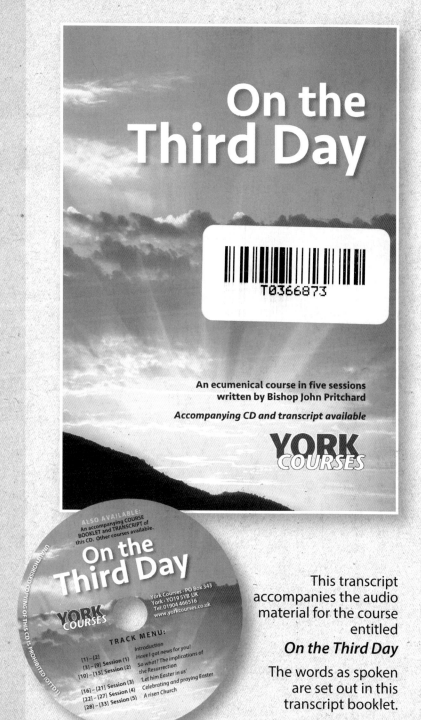

On the Third Day

An ecumenical course in five sessions
written by Bishop John Pritchard

Accompanying CD and transcript available

YORK
COURSES

UNAUTHORISED COPYING OF THIS CD IS PROHIBITED (OTTD1)

ALSO AVAILABLE:
An accompanying COURSE
BOOKLET and TRANSCRIPT of
this CD. Other courses available.

On the Third Day

YORK
COURSES

York Courses · PO Box 343
York · YO19 5YB UK
Tel: 01904 466516
www.yorkcourses.co.uk

TRACK MENU:

[1] – [2]		Introduction
[3] – [9]	Session (1)	Have I got news for you!
[10] – [15]	Session (2)	So what? The implications of the Resurrection
[16] – [21]	Session (3)	'Let him Easter in us'
[22] – [27]	Session (4)	Celebrating and praying Easter
[28] – [33]	Session (5)	A risen Church

This transcript
accompanies the audio
material for the course
entitled
On the Third Day

The words as spoken
are set out in this
transcript booklet.

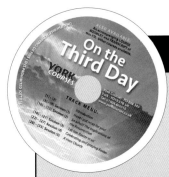

Making full use of the Audio

Index of Track Numbers

[1] – [2]	*Introduction*
[3] – [9] Session (1)	*Have I got news for you!*
[10] – [15] Session (2)	*So what? The implications of the Resurrection*
[16] – [21] Session (3)	*'Let him Easter in us'*
[22] – [27] Session (4)	*Celebrating and praying Easter*
[28] – [33] Session (5)	*A risen Church*

Each track number on the course audio corresponds to the start of each new question posed to the participants by Simon Stanley, the presenter. The track numbers are shown in square brackets in the text of the transcript itself.

When to play the Course Audio

There is no 'right' way! Some groups will play the 14/15-minute piece at the beginning of the session. Other groups do things differently – perhaps playing it at the end, or playing 7/8 minutes at the beginning and the rest halfway through the meeting. The track markers (on the audio and shown in the Transcript) will help you find any question put to the participants very easily, including the Closing Reflections, which you may wish to play (again) at the end of the session. Do whatever is best for you and your group.

COPYRIGHT:

The recorded material and this transcript booklet are covered by the rules of copyright and must not be copied.

© *York Courses:* August 2017

OUR WARM THANKS:

to Katrina Lamb, who transcribed the audio material; to Julie Skelton of Appletree Design Solutions who prepared the artwork; and to Jerry Ibbotson for recording and producing the audio material.

This transcript accompanies the course booklet for
On the Third Day

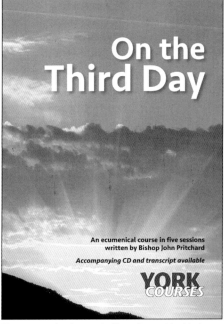

On the Third Day

An ecumenical course in five sessions
written by Bishop John Pritchard

Accompanying CD and transcript available

YORK
COURSES

The image as used on the course booklet, audio material and the front cover of this booklet is copyright © jeka1984 www.istockphoto.com

Full details of our range, including the latest special offers and discounts, are available at www.yorkcourses.co.uk where you can order securely online.

FREE PACKING & SECOND CLASS POST IN THE UK

York Courses presents

ON THE THIRD DAY

York Courses presents
On the Third Day,
a course in five sessions.

CD Track [1]

Hello, I'm Simon Stanley and I'm delighted to be your guide through this course. But before we meet our four distinguished contributors, here's a short introduction by Bishop John Pritchard, the writer of the course booklet on which this audio is based.

JP: I don't know about you, but I'm always disappointed by the short life and early death of Easter. We have a long, strong build-up through the serious weeks of Lent and the dark days of Holy Week. We plumb the depths on Good Friday, hold our breath on Holy Saturday and then explode with delight on Easter Day. But by lunchtime it's all gone. Easter is the ace, king and queen of Christian festivals. It's what our faith is all about. It's the signature tune of Christianity. How can it vanish so soon?

Of course, first of all, we need to be sure of our facts. So the first session in this Lent course looks again at the event of the resurrection, and why we can trust it as solid ground. I know dead men don't rise from the grave – it's outrageous. But that's just the point. Welcome to God's new world!

Session Two says: 'Okay, wonderful, but precisely how does the resurrection give shape and colour to what we believe? Let's examine that if it's so important.' It affects what we believe about Jesus, about the cross, about death, about the world and its welfare – about everything.

Session Three says, 'Okay on the head stuff - what we believe - but so what? How does the resurrection affect what we do as Christians?' If Christianity really is a verb before it's a noun; if it's something we live, day by day, before being something we formulate into doctrines, then let's have a go. What does it mean for our discipleship?

Session Four focuses on prayer and worship, and how we celebrate Easter in church and in our own homes. Our official liturgies do the middle register of our emotions very well, but they don't do either ecstasy or lament particularly well. And Easter is ecstasy. And the joy of it needs to overflow into our praying and worshipping as we travel on through the year.

The last session asks the question: 'If we have a risen Christ, how can we have a risen Church?' That seems a fair question and we'll examine what a risen church might look like in session Five. So, as they used to say on the radio: 'If you're sitting comfortably, then we'll begin …'

[2] *And now let me briefly introduce the contributors to you.*

Paul Vallely is a leading British writer on religion, ethics, Africa and development issues and was a distinguished foreign correspondent for many years. He's a Roman Catholic and wrote the best-selling book 'Pope Francis: Untying the Knots'. Ruth Gee was President of Methodist Conference in 2013/14 and is chair of the Darlington Methodist District and is the Church's representative within Churches Together in England. Tom Wright is a leading international New Testament scholar, a Pauline theologian and a retired Anglican Bishop. He's now Research Professor of New Testament and Early Christianity at the University of St Andrews. Libby Lane was the first woman to become a bishop in the Church of England and is Bishop of Stockport in the Diocese of Chester.

So, introductions over - let's begin!

Session 1 – Have I got news for you!

[3]

The resurrection of Jesus Christ is central to the Christian faith, but faith in the resurrection can take a number of forms. For many Christians it's deeply intuitive - something you sort of just know to be true; while for others it's highly rational, because there's plenty of evidence. I asked our contributors where they stand on this spectrum. First Ruth Gee, then Paul Vallely, and finally Tom Wright.

RG: The rational arguments take me so far, especially the resurrection appearances, but it's also a deeply experienced reality. So the knowledge of God, of the presence of God, I

glimpse the glory of God in so many places. Sometimes it's in the obvious: it might be beautiful mountain scenery, somewhere like Snowdonia. But it's also in the more difficult places: at the bedside of the dying offering hope, or in the midst of tragedy - that deep inner certainty. So for me it's both: the rational arguments, and that inner experience.

PV: For me the resurrection is intuitive. It's part of the mystery - the things that are beyond words. And it's communicated primarily through people - through the acts of people in difficult situations. So for me the resurrection is there in the people who come to the aid and succour of those who are in distress or in need.

TW: Some people really don't mind about the rational arguments. They say: 'if I can sense the presence of the living Jesus, that's quite enough for me.' Other people will say: 'I know this is totally irrational, so you're going to have to convince me that it is in fact the best possible explanation.' And I think the great thing about the gospel is it will stand up to investigation, whichever way you come at it. Not that we ever have Jesus in our pockets. It's important to say that. We can't construct a rational argument which ends up with us saying: 'Therefore, my argument is a + b + c = Resurrection. Therefore you've got to believe it, or you're stupid!' as it were. Because it's always about God doing something huge and different, which is new creation. And the point about that is that it is like the old creation, only a total renewal, so that it's not irrational in that sense, but it is a new sort of way of being in the world which has not happened - in other words, it isn't just a resuscitation; it isn't just a bizarre trick within the old creation. It is the paradigmatic and launching event of the new creation. And for that we need - ultimately a full Christian response would be heart and mind and soul and strength, so the mind and the soul come into that larger category.

[4] *After the resurrection happens you could bump into Jesus anywhere: in a garden, an upper room, on a seashore. I asked our contributors where they bump into the risen Christ most often. Ruth, Paul and Tom.*

RG: Absolutely everywhere. And most often in the most unexpected places. To give just one example, a few years ago I visited Zimbabwe, and in places where there was a lot of hardship and suffering at that time people would come up to me and say: 'God is good'. And glimpsing the risen Christ in those places was both surprising and awe-inspiring.

PV: When people are looking for the resurrected Jesus they're told: 'He is not here. He's not here where you expect him to be. He's not in Jerusalem. He's not in the centre of power and politics. He's gone back to Galilee. Go and seek him in Galilee. Galilee is the place of everyday life. It's a place of fishing and carpentry and, you know, you need to go back there.' So, where do we see the risen Christ? We see him where we don't expect him - not where he used to be, not in the church necessarily, not in the centres of powers, but out in the messy world. And that's where we need to keep our eyes open, because he can come and you can miss him.

TW: I do know that there are some Christians - one chap was talking to me just a few months ago about this, shared with me his own experience of suddenly finding Jesus visibly, physically present with him when he was, I think, in his early twenties or something, and it was a totally life-changing experience, but he knows, and I know, that that is very, very unusual. If you study the literature there are not many people who've had that kind of experience. So for most of us it's a sense of presence - of recognisable presence - but not in that way where the door would actually open and in he would come. And that recognisable presence, as in the Emmaus road story, and it's obviously written in such a way as to say that there are continuities with regular Christian experience through the scriptures and the breaking of bread, the scriptures and the breaking of bread, again and again. I mean, God moves in many mysterious ways. I would never want to set limits to what God can do because, as a pastor, I've heard lots of extraordinary stories. And I just say: 'well, thank you Lord, if that's what you wanted to do with that person'. But I wouldn't want any one to imagine that because they hadn't had one of those exceptionally vivid and senses of the presence of Jesus they were somehow second-rate citizens, because that's certainly not the case.

[5] *In the booklet John Pritchard writes that his faith in the resurrection moved him from a 'don't know' to a joyful 'yes'. But what about those Christians who can't in all honesty say a joyful 'yes' because they're not sure? Paul, Tom and Ruth.*

PV: You don't feel or think the same thing all the time. Faith is a process, it's a journey, and it's not a constant necessarily. And so this idea that, you know, you can be this kind of joyful, positive, clappy person just doesn't touch the pulse of my daily experience. And I think you need to think about faith as a roller-coaster.

TW: I prefer the word 'sureness' to 'certainty' because the word 'certainty' has a kind of a brittle flavour to it, and I think we've all learned that there is a kind of a wrong sort of lust for certainty. And so I would want to say if somebody really has that sense that Jesus, the living Jesus, is a presence to them, I'd say: 'Let's work on firming up on your faith in what actually happened, but let's work on that from within Christian faith' and not saying: 'You're outside until you can sign all these documents on the line.'

RG: I just think of the times when Jesus wasn't sure. Should he help the daughter of a foreign woman, or should he not? And that prayer in Gethsemane: ' if it's possible, take this cup from me'. And the cry that he made from the cross: 'My God, my God, why have you forsaken me?' I may cry out with a joyful 'Yes, Christ is risen indeed!' but sometimes it's more a cry of hope than a cry of certainty. And at those times it's often the on-going liturgy of the Church that will anchor me and sustain me when I can't hope or believe. I'm still a part of the body of people who hold that belief, and sometimes they hold it on my behalf. It doesn't all depend on me. I'm a Christian in the company of others.

[6] *So can those who are not absolutely sure even call themselves Christians?*

TW: Yeah, the question of who we call Christian is a very dangerous one, because it does imply a kind of elitist or - you know, 'we're the real deal and those people over there aren't'. I used to get into trouble because a dear friend of mine, Marcus Borg - Marcus did not believe in the bodily resurrection of Jesus, but he had a very vivid faith in Jesus as a living presence. Clearly, there was a strong sense of the presence of Jesus, and I knew Marcus well enough to think he wasn't fooling himself. The thing was, he had come from a tradition which had basically been very conservative and rationalist, where you just had to believe: Bang! This happened, that happened - so I used to say to him: 'Marcus, as far as I can see you are a Christian, but I think you're a bit muddled on this front.' And he of course would return the compliment.

RG: I think to be a Christian you have to believe that there is life overcoming death, that the light overcomes the darkness, but we're all on a journey to understanding fully what that means. And at points on that journey we will find it more difficult than at other times. So we share in the faith and the hope and the life of all the believers, and we work with that. And I don't think any one of us on our own has all the answers or the faith that's needed.

PV: I think it would be pretty odd to not believe that Jesus rose on the third day because so much of the succour that you draw is from that experience. But no, I think you could be a Christian and not believe in the resurrection, and just be part of the Christian community. I think that's feasible.

[7] *Rowan Williams makes this huge claim about the resurrection: 'When we celebrate Easter we are really standing in the middle of a second Big Bang, a tumultuous surge of divine energy as fiery and intense as the very beginning of the universe.' I asked if this made sense to our contributors. What would a scientist make of it?*

RG: It's a metaphor. But everything we say about God is necessarily metaphor, and science also actually speaks quite often in metaphors. So, I think the conversation with the scientist would be around different ways of understanding truth, different ways of describing truth. And no, of course it's not literally a 'Big Bang', but what we're saying is that in the effect of the resurrection, and the difference it makes to human life, then it's like the Big Bang.

PV: What Rowan's talking about there is the intense fiery transformative power that the resurrection can have inside you. Not always, but sometimes, you're just seized with this conviction and you feel 'yes' and that changes the way that you look at the world. I don't think science is appropriate there.

TW: Many scientists I know say: 'Absolutely as a scientist I study the way the world currently is, but this doesn't say that the world could never have a fresh injection of new creation, a new Big Bang'. So it depends whether the scientist is prepared to say: 'as a scientist I'm going with all the evidence even if it tells me something I wasn't expecting' or whether as a scientist that person would want to say: 'because I can observe the natural world the way it is I have reached the very different conclusion that nothing new can ever

actually happen' and that's actually a metaphysical rather than a scientific position to take.

[8] *So, another way to ask that first question again. Is the resurrection more a mystery to enter into than a fact to dissect on a table?*

PV: Part of the whole business of being a Christian is that you have this intuition that the world is not the bald, reductive, materialist place that some sceptics and scientists and rationalists would have you believe. There is more - there is love, there is poetry, there is ritual, there is deep psychological emotion, all of that is in the resurrection. And to say: 'is the resurrection a fact?' is to diminish the resurrection enormously.

RG: We can talk about the empty tomb, and the evidence for and against the empty tomb. We can talk about the appearances, and people testifying to having met with the risen Christ. There are facts that we can look at. But at the end of the day, yes, it's a mystery. We know that it is not the normal course of events that people who are dead come back to life. There's something mysterious about that. There's something unique about that.

TW: But of course it's a mystery to enter into, because the whole point of it, as in the gospels, is the resurrection is about God launching a new creation, and saying: 'come on in, look what we're doing, you can join in.' And that is a mystery because it is continuous with, but different from, life as it's going on at the moment. It's a mystery in the sense that it's something you enter into by prayer, and it's something you enter into through contemplation and meditation and through serving the work of the gospel, and you discover, as Albert Schweitzer famously said: 'You discover who the risen Jesus is as you move further and further into that mystery'. So it's a lot of both.

[9] *And to end this session, Bishop Libby Lane reflects on the reality of the Resurrection.*

Easter reminds us of the great promise that nothing of our creation will be wasted. Refined, purified, redeemed, made new certainly, but not wasted.

One of the privileges of parish ministry is to be entrusted with the conducting of funeral services. And sometimes I would imagine the truths of the liturgy as a container, in which deep-felt but often hard to articulate responses - grief, anger, confusion, sadness, or relief, thanksgiving, precious memories - can be safely held. The container will not break.

Death, whether sudden or anticipated, generates powerful responses in us, and confronts us with the prospect of our own mortality. In such circumstances, at a time when we are at our most vulnerable, the message of the Resurrection can offer the hope that nothing of the love we have given and received is rendered pointless, thrown back in our faces by the stark fact of death.

Jesus tells us in John 6.39: 'And this is the will of the One who sent me, that I should lose not even one of all that has been given me, but raise them all up on the last day.' Love really is stronger than death. Love raised Jesus from the dead and Love promises the same to us. Nothing will be wasted.

Session 2 – So what? The implications of the Resurrection

[10]

If we read 1 Corinthians Chapter 15 we know with our head that death has been defeated, but how confident are we with our heart in life after death? I asked our contributors. First, Paul Vallely.

PV: You ask the question: 'how confident am I'? Well, it always seems to me that confidence is the enemy of faith. It's too easy. We have confidence in facts. Faith is something that, you know - we're making a leap. We're reaching after something. So, we have these intuitions, and senses of things being there but we're not quite sure what they are. That's what faith is. So 'confident' is not a word I would use.

Now Ruth Gee.

RG: I'm on a journey. I proclaim my faith in life after death and I hold onto it with all honesty. But I have my times of doubt. I have the times when I ask: 'what if death is the absolute end of me?' But I am completely confident that I am loved by God and so perhaps, in the end, I will continue to exist only as one loved eternally by God. But that's not bad.

And Tom Wright.

TW: The New Testament has very little to say about life after death. There's the dying thief on the cross 'today you'll be with me in paradise'. That doesn't last long, because today then Jesus is back again, risen from the dead, leaving the thief in paradise, whatever that means, until the resurrection day. Paul says:

'My desire is to depart and be with the Messiah, which is far better' but then later in Philippians he talks about Jesus coming and transforming our body to be like his glorious body. So there's a two-stage post mortem reality. And in John 14 you have the same thing of Jesus saying: 'In my Father's house there are many dwelling places' but the word for a dwelling place there is not a final resting place, it's not a mansion, as the old translation has it, it's a place you go to be rested and refreshed *until* the day when the resurrection happens. So there's so much confusion about that still, and even though I and others have been banging on about this for some years, people go back into default mode and they think: 'Oh, it's all about life after death'. Well, it's much more interesting than that.

[11] When all is said and done, the cross is a strange kind of victory. I asked Tom how he thinks it works, such an awful death becoming a victory.

TW: The New Testament is quite clear that something happened on the cross which has to be spoken of in terms of victory. And most of the early fathers said that as well, and they weren't stupid. They knew that people still died, that nasty accidents still happened, that sickness was still rife etc. but they went on saying - because Paul says it in Colossians apart from anything else - that on the cross Jesus defeated the principalities and powers. So Jesus is saying that his own forthcoming death will be the time when he claims sovereignty over the whole world, displacing and defeating the one he calls 'the ruler of this world'. Something has happened to liberate people, in principle, people are liberated from the chains of sin and death and they are free to respond to the gospel in a way that wasn't true before. Now, how did that work? In all four gospels they give the answer to that, not as a theory but as mini-narratives. So, in Luke you have Jesus dies but Barabbas goes free. Jesus is innocent, but the thief on the cross is guilty, nevertheless, Jesus promises him a place in paradise etc. There are lots and lots of little stories which are about Jesus dying in the place of others, and so the victory is won through what, in the trade, we might call 'representative substitution'. Because Jesus is the Messiah, he represents his role, he represents the world, therefore he can stand in and take their place. And when Paul is talking about this victory in Romans 8, he says there is no condemnation for those who are in Christ Jesus because dot dot dot on the cross God condemned sin in the flesh. This is where all the theories of atonement come rushing together, and you need the representative substitution to explain the victory. You can't do the one without the other. People have tried and it just doesn't work. In the New Testament you have to have the whole picture together.

[12] Paul offers a rather earthy way of describing the process.

PV: When something bad happens to us, it impacts not just us but the people around us. So, you know, you can be sad, or you can be in a bad mood, and you kind of transmit that to your wife, who thinks, you know, what's the matter with him? And you're kind of passing on some of the pain to your wife. I mean in crude terms it's called 'kick-the-cat' isn't it. You know, you've hit your thumb with a hammer, hammering a nail, and the cat comes by and you kick the cat to get rid of your feelings! You know, we don't do that literally, but we do that metaphorically, and we do that in our general relationships with people. We transmit the pain. We pass it on. What happened at the crucifixion was that Jesus absorbed the pain and he didn't pass it on. And so that process of the abused child becoming an abusing adult, and that cycle going on forever, that that's part of the psychological dynamic of what it is to be a human, and Jesus stopped that. He put a full stop at that. He absorbed the pain into himself and he said: 'Father, forgive them'. So in doing that, he offered us this extraordinary example of how we need to stop kicking the cat. When people forgive, it cures something inside themselves, and people who don't forgive nurse a bitterness that rankles and destroys them. So forgiving, although it's very hard, is something that what we're taught is, it will help us. It doesn't just help the person who's forgiven, it helps the forgiver. It helps the forgiver go forward in life in a creative and positive way, rather than going forward in an embittered and chewed-up way.

[13] *John Pritchard writes in the booklet 'because of the resurrection we've glimpsed the goal of history, journey's end, the new creation. In the middle of history the end has begun.' I asked Ruth and Tom what they think that end is. Could they give any first sketches of this new world?*

RG: I no longer in my imagination see a physical place. I think of relationships, and being in the presence of God and in the presence of others, and in some way that's localised, but I think it's - the locality is, the presence of God. And I know that sounds vague, and unsatisfactory for some I'm sure, but that is how I imagine it and envision it as being: in the presence of God, in relationship with others, transcending all the messy bits and the particularities of human relationships as I know them now.

TW: The New Jerusalem and all that therein is. It's as though these are different ways of saying: 'Because we know little bits about how human life works now, we can extrapolate forwards and say it will be something like the great final victory at the end of a terrible battle. It will be something like the new birth, you know, a new child at last, and something like a glorious wedding of bride and groom who've waited for a long time and finally this is it.' Only, of course, all those writers would want to say: 'these are just signposts.' I've often said: 'All our language about the future is a set of signposts pointing into a fog.' They're true signposts, but they don't give you more than a glimmer, a symbol of what it's actually going to be like when you get there.

[14] *To say Christ is alive, and can be known as a friend, can sound very presumptuous. What does it mean? Paul first, then Ruth and Tom.*

PV: This is not the kind of language that I would use: 'Jesus is my friend'. It kind of - it's too direct, and it smacks of the literal. Because it means, like, you know, 'my best friend, the person I went to school with, the person I go out for a drink with'. That is not how

I have a relationship with Christ. It is much more atmospheric, tangential; it's more indirect - it's more like being in the presence of somebody. You present to Jesus in his presence the problems you're having, or the inadequacies that you detect in yourself when you are being honest, and it's a situation in which that kind of stripping-away can happen, and you can be more ruthless about your own self and your own inadequacies. And that's kind of, in the atmosphere of, in the presence of, rather than 'I tell Jesus this story and/or make this confession to him of something that I've done and then he gives me an answer'. Because prayer doesn't work like that for me. You don't get the answer in a form of words, to a question in a form of words. When you get an answer in prayer it's an insight or a resolution, and you feel, 'yes, now I know'. And all of that is much more vague than talking to a friend and getting a direct answer.

RG: The heart of it is that it means that I am never alone; even when I feel lonely and isolated, I'm simply not alone. And one of the things that comes to my mind when I'm asked this question is a card that's on the windowsill of somebody I know very well, which simply says: 'Lord, help me to remember that there is nothing that will happen today that you and I can't handle together.' And that's what it is for me. It's that knowledge that I'm not alone. That there is always somebody there with me.

TW: As a pastor I've met people who have had faithful, prayerful, worshipping lives but to whom it comes as a real shock to think of Jesus as a friend. And they think that's a bit blasphemous: 'Could I really say that?' And when I was working with students I would find people who would be really nervous about that, at the same time as other people who had only ever thought of Jesus as a friend, from their tradition, and were having to face the fact that friendships change and develop, and that they may need to grow up a bit and have a more mature relationship.

[15] And now our closing reflection by Libby.

I was asked recently about Resurrection. What, precisely, was resurrected? Jesus' skin and bones, giving him a recognizable physiognomy? His muscles, giving him movement? His digestive system? His heart and lungs?

The tomb, according to the Gospel accounts, was empty. No physical traces left. They also report that the risen Jesus was not immediately recognisable to his followers. He did however share meals with them, and cooked breakfast on the shore of Galilee. When Thomas pressed his fingers against Jesus's flesh, the wounds were still there. His fingers didn't pass through as if Jesus were a ghost.

I think perhaps I was having the wrong conversation, or at least only part of the right conversation. The resurrection is about why, as much about how and what. The problem with solely physical speculations is that they draw us into thinking about the Resurrection as a 'reanimation' - a jolting into life of dead cells which appear to regain their former functions, with some added features. This is to view the action of God from within the sealed world of human experience.

The Resurrection is real - indeed more real than our human understanding of reality. But it is also a 'new thing' - an irruption of grace and love into a world in need of mercy, unable to supply it for itself.

Session 3: 'Let him Easter in us' – Personal discipleship in the light of the Resurrection.

[16]

If it's true, as John Pritchard writes in his booklet, that 'the world rests in the purposes of God', does it mean that God would stop us blowing ourselves up - or irrevocably damaging the planet through global warming? It's a question I put to our contributors Paul Vallely, Ruth Gee and Tom Wright.

PV: Part of the glory of being made in the image of God is that we've been given freedom. We've been given freedom to - and freedom involves the ability to do the wrong thing as well as the choice to do the right thing, and we have consistently done the wrong thing through history, we know that. It's too, kind of, prescriptive a notion to talk about the purpose of God for the world, as though it's a kind of scientific formula – like, at the end of an experiment you write 'Conclusion'. So therefore God wants this, and we have to find ways of understanding and embracing that, even if we can't spell it out literally. So 'the purposes of God', I think, is something which is much more profound than you'd get from a kind of historical or scientific explanation.

RG: God's purposes aren't confined to this planet, to this short space of time in all eternity. The wonder is that we can glimpse God's purposes here and now, but the fulfilment of those purposes is of a completely different order, and won't be derailed even if we do blow ourselves up or irrevocably damage the planet. I'm not saying that God is planning it that way, I'm saying that that is a possibility within the life that we live and within the freedoms that God allows us.

TW: People often say: 'why did God allow this or that or the other to happen?' You know, after a terrible road accident, 'Why did God let that happen?' The answer is, do you want God, every time somebody tries to take a corner too fast, to suspend the laws of physics and say: 'No, no, we can't have that'. You know, in other words, to keep us in cotton wool. God has given humans responsibility, much more than most of us realise actually, and having done that, God wants us to exercise that responsibility. At the same time I would say, just like the security services tell us that: 'We're not giving you any details but actually 55 terrorist plots have been foiled by the security services over the last two years', or whatever it is, I would be perfectly prepared to believe that over the last five minutes, five years, five centuries, God has in fact stopped us doing all kinds of crazy things. And that maybe God allows us to feel the effects of our folly thus far and no further.

[17] *John Pritchard writes, 'we mustn't over-claim our faith, making out that it's always a wonderful champagne-and-strawberries experience'. But why isn't it?*

TW: There are moments, I think, when there are times of great joy which are far beyond champagne and strawberries. But at the same time, in the New Testament it's quite clear that the way the victory of the cross is implemented in the world is through God's people sharing the sufferings of the Messiah. Paul is very explicit; Peter is very explicit - in 1st Peter - writing to people who might have thought: 'well, Jesus did the suffering bit, so can we have the joy now please'. And Peter has to say: 'Don't be surprised that you have to go through this as well. This is how the gospel makes its way in the world'. And it always has. The victory which was achieved through suffering has to be implemented through suffering. The good news is that Paul onwards, in the early Christian tradition - suffering and joy seem to go very closely together, and the people who have that intense suffering sometimes speak also of a joy which far transcends anything else. And I hesitate to speak of that, as I say, because I'm not somebody who's suffered a great deal, but I believe the testimony of the people who've said that.

RG: Human life involves things that can go wrong, relationships that can go wrong, the ageing of our bodies and minds, and illness and pain, alongside the life-giving relationships and pleasures and health and vitality. It was like this for Jesus too, and faith is what sustains us in those things. It doesn't make us something other than human.

[18] *John Pritchard asserts that the Resurrection means that we are to bear with one another's foibles and forgive each other. But how do we do that? Is it just a matter of trying harder and harder? I asked our contributors.*

RG: I believe that we can only do it with the help of God, and through the grace of God. But we have to be careful here as well I think, because there are also matters of justice and the need to protect those who are abused - in whatever way that might happen. There are some behaviours that we have to challenge and not just bear with, and we have to resist them because they're harmful and wrong. So forgiveness without repentance is what Dietrich Bonhoeffer called 'cheap grace' and that's not the grace of God. So, yes we have to bear with one another's foibles and forgive each other, but that's not just a matter of forgetting, of overlooking, it's also a matter sometimes of challenging.

PV: There's more to it than just 'trying harder'. You have to try and look at the world in a different way. And Pope Francis came up with a good example of this. He said: 'when you give to a beggar, do you look into his eyes? Because if you just toss the money into his cup and walk past, that's a very diminished act of charity, because you're not actually relating to that person as a human being.' And so 'trying harder' to me smacks of throwing more money into more coins. Whereas what it ought to do is say: 'stop, think, look at the world in a different way. Is this how Jesus would look at the world?' And then test yourself against that. And so it's about changing your perception, not about changing your actions.

TW: I was talking to somebody who had been really badly hurt and offended by somebody else behaving in a very bad way to them, and it had been, I don't know how many years - three, four, five years - and they'd been praying for that other person without any sense that 'I want to forgive them', actually 'I still want to punch them on the nose', and then one day, suddenly meeting them unexpectedly, found that they were able to go up and say: 'Hello and how are you?' and talk about this and that, and to come away feeling: 'Oh my goodness, I seem to have forgiven them. How did that happen?' And actually having no resentment at all. It isn't just trying harder and harder, though that - you're going to have to do that too - but that praying for them and with them, so that then, it may be five minutes, it may be five years, forgiveness can and does happen.

[19] *St Paul writes in 1 Corinthian Chapter 15: 'If only for this life we have hope in Christ, we are of all people most to be pitied.' I asked Paul and Ruth if they are afraid of dying.*

PV: The footballer Rio Ferdinand, his wife died of cancer; she was very young - about 28, I think - and he made a TV programme about it. And one of the things he said was that, you know, 'when you're a footballer, all you think about is winning. That is the only thing. So I thought about, you know, how we're going to beat her disease and that was the wrong thing to think.' And he said he thought his wife was perhaps trying to get him to talk about this more, and he didn't want to talk about certain things, and he said: 'now that she's dead, I wonder what she would have wanted to say to our daughter on her 18th birthday. I wonder what she would have wanted to say to my son when he'd got

his university place. I wonder what she …' And he had this, kind of, list of things which he couldn't imagine what she would have said, and he wished he'd asked her. And I think that being afraid of death is part of all of that. So, you can have a kind of spiritual confidence that, you know, you'll be with God; and you'll have some understanding of the cosmic things that you just cannot comprehend; and you can have even the old schoolboy notion of being in a place that is heaven and - but none of those really can answer the kind of psychological angst that comes around the idea of me not being here any more.

RG: I don't want to die, and I don't look forward to the process of dying. I'm afraid of a painful death, and I'm afraid of the sorrow that comes with bereavement. But I'm not afraid of death, because I don't think it's the thing most greatly to be feared. I don't think that death is the worst thing that can happen to me. And so I believe that, even in death, the risen Christ will be with me. So, I might fear the process. I might fear the results of death, and of dying, but death itself – no, I don't fear death itself.

[20] *I wondered if their Christian faith helped them to make sense of life.*

RG: It does, because it means that God is at the centre of all things and not me. And so it gives me a focus point and a direction. It means that when I come across issues in life, when I come across problems, when I have to make decisions, I try to see it from the point of view of God, and not just my point of view. And as I believe that God is at the foundation of all life - the Creator - then that makes sense of life for me.

PV: I can think of a time when I was in a refugee camp, and I was interviewing a woman who had arrived and she had a child who didn't look very well at all, in the hospital, and they'd travelled, and they'd left her husband with one child, who was too sick, back home. They would come to get the food, and they were going to take it back. So she didn't know what had happened to her husband or her other child. She had a third child who'd died on the journey there. At the end of this process, and I said to the translator to say, 'Thank you very much. That's all the information I need, thank you. And I hope that her child gets better'. And then the woman said something, and I said to the translator: 'What did she say?' And she said: 'The woman said: "How many children do you have? And how old are they? And how well are they?"' And I looked at this woman, who had been an object to me, an object in a story, a character in a play. And she looked at me, and I saw something in her eyes which I - afterwards I would have said, looking at it from a Christian point of view, was that I saw Christ in her.

TW: Life throws all kinds of things at you. Being a Christian, yes, it does help, but making sense creeps up on you from behind. It isn't just working out a mathematical formula. However, I've studied and taught the whole question of world views: how world views work, the stories we tell, the symbols we use, the habitual practices we have, the instinctive answers we give to obvious big questions - who am I? Where am I? What's wrong? What's the solution? What time is it? I've kind of thought all that through. That still wouldn't necessarily help when really bad things happen. But then that sense, at every point of the presence of God in Christ, whether it's in worship in the church, in Eucharist, whether it's in daily prayer, whether it's in scripture readings, whatever, in the faces and company of Christian friends, brothers and sisters, that is a total making sense for me. So yeah, but it isn't just: 'Oh, I'm a Christian, therefore I can think solo up into some sort of making sense. It's much more interesting than that.'

[21] *And we now turn to Libby again for her closing reflection.*

There is a wonderful sonnet by Gerard Manley Hopkins called *God's Grandeur*. At first it sorrows over the desecration of the earth, and the reduction of God's grand shining creation to a bleary, smoky world, made ashen by humanity. But then Hopkins finds a new hope below the cindered crust: 'There lives the dearest freshness deep down things...' and although the sun has set in the west, a new morning sun rises eastward: 'Because the Holy Ghost over the bent / World broods with warm breast and with ah! bright wings.'

The poem reminds me that the Resurrection involves the whole of creation. To live in its light means not just undergoing personal renewal but rethinking and reforming our relationship with the earth. Rather than discarding creation like a dead skin, we recognise that it is 'charged with the Grandeur of God' and treasure it as a precious gift which speaks of the generosity as well as the glory of God.

The poem also offers hope: the 'freshness' survives from the actions of the Holy Spirit. We are sustained by the same Spirit, the Comforter and Advocate whom Jesus sent to the world, and who breathes freshness and energy and joy into us too, awakening the deepest part of ourselves and encouraging us to walk lightly and sustainably within the Kingdom.

Session 4 – Celebrating and praying Easter

[22]

We pray frequently to an almighty God, but do we pray enough to a gentle God or even a terrifying God? I asked Paul Vallely and Ruth Gee whether the Resurrection might feed into, maybe energise or inform our praying.

PV: I think the Resurrection does change the way - must change the way that we pray, because the resurrection means that God is a man: Jesus. It's easier to pray to someone who you feel has an intuitive understanding because he has shared the situations that you're in. If you were praying without Jesus, you'd be, you know, you'd try to plug yourself into the wider cosmic consciousness, or whatever. That kind of God - it would be very hard to pray to.

RG: I do remember one night going to bed feeling absolutely empty, and feeling that I was in the wrong place, that I couldn't possible be called by God, and waking up in the night, and the experience there - I fell asleep praying - was of being enfolded in a very warm blanket and just being sure that it was okay. So that was a gentle and life-affirming experience. At other times I've prayed and been absolutely convinced through prayer that God has wanted me to go and enter into a particular situation that really I would prefer not to. But that that was what I needed to

do and had to do, and I've had to follow that through. And it hasn't always been easy, but God has been there with me in it.

[23] *The Benedictines endeavour to receive guests as though they were receiving Christ. I wondered what difference it would make if we all followed that rule.*

PV: I don't think most of us, in our busy lives, have got time to do that. It's an ideal. And when Pope Francis says, 'if you give to a beggar you should look into his eyes' I think he's hinting at that, which is that you have to see Christ in everybody. And ideally one would have the time to stop and do that, and have the mind shift to do that. The reality of the way we live our lives is that we can only do that occasionally, and it has to be a kind of mental paradigm shift. But, I think if you were consumed by the consciousness of that on a daily basis with everybody you met, you'd either be a saint - or you'd be overwhelmed.

RG: At the very least, for a Christian, it must mean receiving people with respect, and receiving them as an honoured guest - somebody we really want to be with. Somebody who we are really prepared to listen to, and receive as they are. Somebody that we really believe we might be able to learn something from. No, not might, that we *will* be able to learn something from. Somebody we really value. Somebody who we're going to put first. Their comfort is going to be more important to us than our own. And if all that's true then we're going to be less inclined to be self-centred as we meet with, and receive, other people. So for a Christian that's what it must mean surely to receive Christ: to receive other people, as if we're receiving Christ.

TW: I think it would make a huge difference. C S Lewis says somewhere: 'you have never met a mere mortal' - I'm paraphrasing it in other words, because, particularly if it's your Christian neighbour, then Christ lives in that person. And, he has a lovely line, something about 'the people we work with, joke with, marry, snub, exploit, these people are actually extraordinary creatures who we should be in awe of'. Now, you can't actually go through your life being in awe of every single person on the street, but there's a proper deep, rich human respect, which ought to be there for everyone.

[24] *How can we learn to practise the presence of the risen Christ? Paul, Ruth and Tom offer some ideas.*

PV: 'Practise the presence.' I'm not sure what 'practise the presence' means. To me, 'be in the presence' is the better phrase, and you can be in the presence of Christ in a way which concentrates your mind and which you focus your full attention on. Only occasionally. You couldn't do it all the time unless you were, you know, a full-time contemplative, or saint.

RG: There's a lot of emphasis today on mindfulness, and that's something that Christians have always regarded as being an essential - to be in the present moment and to recognise that Christ is in it with us and then to try and view things and experience things in the company of Christ. So an example might be that if I'm chairing a difficult meeting, then sometimes I might have a holding cross in my hand, and just holding that cross in my hand helps me to focus on what's important about that situation and that time, that it is that we are in the presence of Christ and that we are - it's usually a Christian meeting - that we're trying to be Christians together here, and so that's about being in the presence of the living Christ in that experience.

TW: In the Ignatian tradition they suggest taking specific stories from scripture and consciously imagining the scene, with yourself as a character on the edge. So the two on the road to Emmaus - just, let's just walk three or four paces behind and listen in on this conversation, and then wait for the moment as you're imagining it and taking time over that, when Jesus might just turn round and beckon and, you know, 'come on up and join us, we're having an interesting chat here' and see what he says to you. And the people who've done spiritual direction, on either side of the table as it were, on that basis will say that that is very often a very, very fruitful, a disturbingly fruitful thing. Certainly, when I've recommended to people that they do that, the stories that they come back with are really quite striking. Where they got down into the story, and at a certain point Jesus turned and noticed them, and said something and invited them - whatever. But this isn't for everybody. There are different pathways because we're all such different personalities. It can become artificial, but it can be ways of discerning who we are, in order that an understanding of ourselves may be present with the Jesus whom we're invoking. And that's something which does take wise direction very often, but anyone can start at any time, and Jesus is there waiting for it to happen.

[25] *John Pritchard talks about 'solar spirituality': full of the joy and glory of Easter, and about 'lunar spirituality'. Our contributors explain the contrasts and what 'lunar spirituality' might look like.*

PV: The Church traditionally, through the centuries, talked about *mysterium lunae*, the 'mystery of the moon', and that was in the sense that the moon doesn't have any light - it reflects the light of the sun. And the mystery of the Church is that it reflects the light of Christ. In the session before the vote in which he was elected, Pope Francis made mention of *mysterium lunae* and said: 'the Church mustn't fool itself that it has a light of its own'. He talked about a self-referential Church - that was the danger. A Church which believes it has its own light. So to me the idea of a 'lunar spirituality' is one which kind of faces up to the fact that we have to kind of get rid of this self-delusion that we have any light.

RG: For me this is about being in the darkness with only the dimly reflected light of the sun, because the moon does that. It reflects the light of the sun for us. But even that very small disturbance of the dark promises that the sun is still there, and that the sun will rise again in the morning. I think that's what it means to me - a 'lunar spirituality', it's that spirituality where we live in the sure and certain hope that the sun will rise.

TW: I was listening on the radio just this morning; for some reason Radio 3 played the *Magnificat & Nunc Dimittis* from Howells' Gloucester Service. Now it's interesting, because Howells himself struggled with belief, and I think would say he wasn't – would have said he was not really a Christian believer. But he glimpsed enough. And he put some of the glory into his music. And when they're singing, 'Glory be to the Father and the Son and the Holy Spirit' at the end of the *Magnificat & Nunc Dimittis* there is a moment of absolute transcendent glory, where the treble will suddenly swoop up to a note, and I almost had to stop the car - I mean [*laughs*] I can't sing the treble note, but I almost had to stop the car and just give thanks for that. And I wasn't expecting it, I was just driving to work, as you do, and suddenly this moment of reflective glory comes and just hits you. And I have to say, he himself had glimpsed enough of that to be able to put that into the music. So whether that was astral or lunar or whatever, I don't know. So, yeah, it's there, it's possible. But I think, for most people, the normal way of a 'lunar spirituality' would be through other people - through being with people who quietly reflect the light.

[26] *John Pritchard suggests that Easter fades far too quickly and needs rescuing. Our contributors are not all sure that's the case, but some have ideas about how it may get a higher profile.*

PV: I don't accept this idea that Easter fades too quickly. You know, it's apt. There's a moment, which is the intense moment of Easter, and then we get back to the everyday. And it's part of the cycle - the Church calendar, you know. We're confident that Easter will come back next year, as it will come back every time there is a resurrection moment. And that can happen, you know, many times a day and not just once a year. It's good to have Easter there as a, kind of, moment - but you wouldn't want to try and, you know, maintain that all of the time. And that's why we have a Church calendar, because we have this kind of, you know, roller-coaster of events. And that reflects the roller-coaster of life, I think.

RG: I think we often rush through our major festivals and major celebrations - Christmas *and* Easter. We think of them as being one-day events, and they're not. They're so much more than that. So we need to take very seriously the fact that Eastertide begins on Easter Day and continues through to Pentecost. We have a whole season of rejoicing. And we have every Sunday throughout the rest of the year of celebrating Easter. So we need to keep the symbols of Easter prominent in our churches and in our homes throughout that time. Not just for the weekend, but for the whole of that season.

TW: Finding creative ways of doing fresh things - that's what Easter ought to be about. Now, as the backup of that, I've said often enough, of course we should have champagne for breakfast on Easter Day, and of course we should have it at least every day during Easter Week. I once did that at home – absolutely shocked my children when they realised Dad really meant it - we're going to be having champagne for breakfast all week! And - but for goodness sake, if this is a new bubbly life, why not actually do things, even if they're a bit silly things, which say: 'we are celebrating the fact that new creation has been launched, even in the middle of this sad old world'. And if we only just sort of, say it for one day and then go away and stop saying it, then it really looks as if we don't mean it.

[27] *And so we turn again to Libby Lane for her closing reflection.*

Scientists who study the world's ancient climates and atmospheres tell us that natural wildfire was a major force in shaping landscape and increasing biodiversity. Studying geological and fossil records gives important clues to the mix of gases and electrical forces that generated widespread burning of vast tracts of vegetation. Over time, species slowly adapted to find ways not only of surviving but thriving in such conditions. Was it the particular mixture of gases that caused vegetation to flourish and become susceptible to burning, or was it the vegetation that created the atmospheric conditions that generated fire?

Perhaps we could think of wildfire as an image of Easter prayer that expresses the interactions of God's Spirit with our human concerns: a refining fire that shapes us and makes us stronger and more resilient, producing new growth and abundant flowering and fruitfulness. It is also the Spirit that prays in us with groans and sighs beyond words - like the crackling of burning timber - which rises to heaven and glorifies the risen Lord. Best of all, it reveals us for who we really are: for burning vegetation, over aeons of geological pressure, hide a carboniferous treasure in its darkness.

To use another image from the poet Gerard Manley Hopkins: 'I am all at once what Christ is, since he was what I am ... immortal diamond.'

Session 5 – A risen Church

[28]

The atheist philosopher Nietzsche wrote: 'I might believe in the Redeemer if his followers looked more redeemed.' I wondered whether our contributors thinks the Church comes across to non-believers as full of Easter life and joy.

RG: I wonder what it looks like to look 'redeemed'. I think that looking redeemed might perhaps be about being people who offer life to others - and we will do that in all sorts of ways. And sometimes it will be about weeping with others and being with them when they go through difficult times. And sometimes it will be about acting for the good of others. As long as we understand looking redeemed to be a very broad category, then yes, I think the Church does often look that way. Sadly, sometimes it doesn't.

TW: He put his finger on something there, that if the Church is really just a religious form of Platonism - in other words the only thing that matters is my disembodied soul and whether it will get to a disembodied heaven - then, of course you may have to chastise yourself and beat yourself up in the present and be a bit miserable about it, because what counts is this future disembodied thing. But Nietzsche was wrong. Christianity isn't Platonism for the masses. Christianity is about new heavens and new earth. And where you see that happening, and thank God it is happening, in the Church of England, in bits of the Scottish Church which I know now, but in plenty of other parts of the world, then it is full of life and joy. And I think even Nietzsche would have noticed that if somebody had drawn his attention to it.

PV: I think ordinary people look at the Church and think it's a weird place. Pope Francis said something like: 'Christians must stop looking like they've just come from a funeral'. There's a sense in which the kind of - the confidence and joy that you get in a lot of Christian circles feels artificial to outsiders, and they look at the Church and the way it treats women, or gay people, or whatever, and think, no, it doesn't seem to be consonant with the message of love and embrace and compassion. It's small daily acts of kindness which will correct the impression that we are on the one hand smug, or on the other hand that we're hypocrites, because we say one thing and then we treat people, even inside the Church, in such different ways. I saw a sign in America which said: 'This church is full of hypocrites - but we can squeeze one more in.'

[29] *That's very comforting, but it still too often feels that change is so very slow in coming in the Church of God. I asked our contributors whether they see signs of resurrection in the Church in the UK and elsewhere.*

PV: The Church will solve its current problems in the way that it's solved the problems of the Reformation - largely by setting them aside. People don't think that the issues for which Catholics and Protestants burned one another in the Reformation are important anymore. They're worried about other things. And there will come a time when people have stopped worrying about the things that we are consumed about, and they'll move on to something else. So, history won't, kind of, resolve itself and it'll all be happily ever after. The process of birth and death, crucifixion and resurrection, will carry on. And what

Jesus is doing through his death, and through his resurrection, is reminding us of that and telling us to apply that all the time. It's not a one-off event. It's a way we need to see the world, and act in the world.

RG: I see signs of resurrection wherever Christians offer healing and hope among themselves and in their community. I see it in small churches and in big ones, in the centre of towns and cities, and in the more rural places. I see it in places where churches work together for the common good. And I see it where Christians stand together against discrimination and violence and injustice, and when we speak out against policies which stigmatise and punish those who are in poverty.

TW: Change is always difficult. The older you get, the harder it is. The habits that we form, form us, and so on. I just got rapped over the knuckles because I've been to the dental hygienist; and she knows perfectly well that however many times she tells me I've got to floss and do this and that and the other, I'm going to be sporadic at best, because the way I clean my teeth is the way I've always cleaned my teeth. And it's actually reasonable effective, and I'm of an age where I think: 'oh go on, you know, do I really need to do this?!' And when we suggest changes in the Church, I see exactly the same reaction. People say: 'oh well, we'll humour him, because we quite like him, sort of, and we'll try it a bit but actually we're not really going to change what we do.' And so, it is very difficult. And God needs to rattle our cages and get us out of that. So, it's always difficult for everybody. However, resurrection does happen. I've seen it. I've seen churches where hardly

anybody went and then when there was a chance to put a new priest in there - sometimes it took two years of people praying and agonising: 'who shall we get and what should we be doing?' and then, in an unexpected way, suddenly, something happens. The right person emerges at last. People have been praying, often for a long time. New life springs up. And when you see that, it's unmistakable. You just think: 'well we've been praying about this a long time, so these new shoots which are coming here, this is the work of God's Spirit, there's no question about it.'

[30] *According to John Pritchard, Easter Christians will want to be involved in the whole warp and weft of our social fabric, affirming life and wanting to make the world better. Are we life-affirming? Or are we too dominated by rules and tradition?*

PV: Well, the answer is both. We're all capable of being both, and of oscillating between the two. And so what we're called to, is trying to kind of be honest about ourselves in the presence of God, in prayer, and when we have achieved a new insight, a new discernment, a new knowledge about ourselves, we'll be in a better position to scrutinise and know when we're being life-affirming, and when we're being too dominated by hidebound rules.

TW: Imagine living in a world where there were no rules. We need rules. We need traditions. They are the way that help us live our lives. However, of course, then we can get stuck in that and we can - there are many, many situations where many of the little rules that we make need to be bent or broken, because they're simply conventions, so there's no morals about it. Of course, the moral rules really, really, really matter. They are basically the recipe for living life without damaging ourselves and one another and God's creation. And if anyone thinks: 'oh well, I can ignore this one or that one', then watch out. However, again, we make all kinds of silly rules about how we do stuff in church, and some - it may have been a good idea for somebody some time - but we do need to take them out and dust them off and say: 'could we be doing this differently? Should we be?' There are all sorts of ways in which this is already happening. And I can hear Paul in 1st Thessalonians 4 saying: 'yes, you are already doing it. I just want you to do it more and more please.'

[31] *How different do you think the Church of the year 2030 will be?*

PV: The Church will change its issues, and it will do that in response to some of its own agenda, but also the agenda of the society in which it exists. But the mess of idealism and hypocrisy which constitutes the Church will continue. And Christ's model of crucifixion and resurrection is there for the Church to constantly use to try and get out of that mess. We never will - but we have to keep trying.

RG: I hope it will be different in the way in which the faith is proclaimed, and that that will be relevant for that time and those places. I hope that it will continue to be reshaped for mission that that the essential core of faith in the risen Christ will shine through. And I hope and pray that we will be truly ecumenical, or at least further along the path to that.

TW: I am very hopeful. And partly because I really do believe that the risen Jesus is not finished with his Church. Partly because I have seen, at the grass roots level, so many signs of hope. And when I think of people, formed in those little local communities, growing up - and with that sense that the Gospel actually works. This is not some silly idea that somebody's had, which I'm just going through the motions of - it actually transforms lives. And as long as that's going on, which it is, then I am full of hope. Part of the trouble is, it seems to work mostly on a slow time-scale, but that's not necessarily always going to be the case. There are some people saying: 'if church attendance goes on dwindling the way it's been doing, then all the major denominations are going to face serious financial and managerial crises within the next generation.' If that happens, that doesn't mean God is dead, it means that God is moving on, which God does from time to time. We may not like it, but we have to be prepared for that. You know, in a sense if he's saying: 'time to move on' then there will be things which I will regret leaving behind. But if that is so, so be it.

[32] *Which are the key issues in society where the Christian voice needs to be heard, and could be more effective?*

PV: We have, to kind of, come across not as happy-clappy, or as deeply pious, or as hidden away in reflective monasteries, or whatever. We have to come across as being part of the world like everybody else. Being normal, but in a kind way. I think, you know, if we can do that, we'll have done something.

RG: The Christian voice has to be heard where there's prejudice, where there's discrimination, where people are being prevented from living full human lives by policies that are unjust. That's where the Christian voice has to be heard. And Christians have to be seen to be involved in things like food banks, and things like street pastors - the Christian voice has to be in those places. And we have to be responding and thinking about the challenges of migration and globalisation, and the effects of that; and what that means and how we - how we relate to it. We have to be engaging in those wider issues, all the time.

TW: Getting involved in politics and social action, of course, and that's messy, it's difficult, we won't always get it right – but, where would we be in the world without the William Wilberforces, without the Martin Luther Kings? You know, these are the people who have had the courage to say: 'no, I'm not going away, I'm just going to go on banging on about this until we do something about it.' Some of us campaigned, fifteen years ago, eighteen years ago, about the dropping of international debt - around the time of the millennium. We haven't done enough of it yet – but, that was Christians actually often having fun: having great rallies and singing songs and being cheerful about it - not being long-faced about it, because this is about jubilee, it's about liberty, it's about God doing new things in real communities.

[33] *So, for the last time, we hear from Bishop Libby with her final reflection.*

On the North West coast of the Scottish Highlands there is a small rocky bay, not much more than a cleft in the cliffs, which forms a natural harbour where the Irish saint, Brendan, is believed to have sheltered during his wanderings. Piled up on the shore between the cliffs is layer upon layer of rounded pebbles, forged in the unimaginable pressure of the volcanic earth, and smoothed by the hammering of the ocean over millennia. As the water meets the shore, the stones glisten, and it is easy to think of them as alive with the *shekinah* - the glory of God.

In the hand, close up, you can see the rings of different minerals forced together. Each stone tells its history - of heat and flow and constant change. Each one is particular, different from its neighbour. In former times locals built their houses - and their churches - from these stones.

The worldwide church today was forged in the heat of the resurrection, shaped by the Holy Spirit in the context of the flux and flow of continuing human history. If we look closely, we will see the marks of that formation: imperfections, knocks and cracks, testimony to resilience through time; beauty as the transforming Holy Spirit glistens within words and actions.

Brendan, the sea-faring saint, knew very well the importance of each stone finding its place in community with others, as the Church waits with a longing for the return of her creator.

The Course Booklet...

...is written by **Bishop John Pritchard,** Chair of SPCK and author of 16 books on aspects of Christian belief and practice. He was the House of Lords' lead Bishop on education from 2010 to 2014.

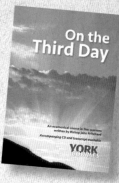

On the Third Day

An ecumenical course in five sessions written by Bishop John Pritchard
Accompanying CD and transcript available

YORK COURSES

PARTICIPANTS on the Course Audio

CANON SIMON STANLEY co-founder of *York Courses* interviews the participants. He is a Canon Emeritus of York Minster and a former BBC producer/presenter.

RT REVD TOM WRIGHT was Bishop of Durham from 2003 to 2010 and is now Research Professor of New Testament at St Andrews. He has written over 80 books and lectured widely around the world.

PROFESSOR PAUL VALLELY writes and lectures on ethics, religion and international development. A director of *The Tablet*, Paul writes for the *New York Times, the Guardian, the Sunday Times* and the *Church Times.*

REVD RUTH GEE is a former President of the Methodist Conference, and is Chair of the Darlington District, and also of the Methodist Council and Moderator of the Churches Together in England Forum.

RT REVD LIBBY LANE became the Church of England's first woman bishop in 2015. Bishop Libby currently serves as Chair of the Diocesan Board of Education, as Chair of the Foxhill Retreat Centre and as Vice-Chair of The Children's Society.

9 781909 107205

York Courses
PO Box 343
York YO19 5YB UK
T: 01904 466516
www.yorkcourses.co.uk
E: info@yorkcourses.co.uk

YORK COURSES

ISBN 978-1-909107-20-5